CBD Oil

Discover How You Can Improve Your Health by Using CBD Hemp Oil With Simple And Effective Methods

this book.

By reading this document, the reader agrees that under no circumstances are is the author responsible for any losses, direct or indirect, which are incurred as a result of the use of information contained within this document, including, but not limited to, —errors, omissions, or inaccuracies.

Table Of Contents

Introduction

The ever-growing cannabis oil industry has led to the discovery of a new category of products which are slowly but surely gaining in popularity. The product category that we are talking about is CBD Hemp Oil.

CBD Hemp Oil or Cannabidiol Oil is becoming increasing popular for use as an effective treatment for a variety of diseases and health disorders. You can see and hear people across the country (and the world) using CBD Hemp Oil in various ways, including but not limited to:

- Putting a few drops into their morning and/or nighttime tea/coffee
- Swallowing capsules
- Inhaling it through their vaping pen
- Putting a drop or two under their tongue
- Applying it topically

The good thing about CBD Oil is that although it is extracted from cannabis plants, it does not get people high (more about this in the next chapter). This is the reason why CBD Hemp Oil is not really popular among users of pot and drugs.

CBD Oil is available in online stores and in retail brick-and-mortar stores as well. The companies that make CBD Hemp Oil will happily deliver it to your doorstep if you choose to order online. Moreover, you can also make CBD Hemp Oil at home, which is a great way to ensure you have it in the purest possible form without having to worry about hidden side-effect-inducing additives.

CBD Oil or Cannabidiol is a compound occurring naturally in the plant species, Cannabis sativa L. Research work conducted in this realm offers promising results based on which medical professionals are encouraged to prescribe it for various ailments, including as an anti-inflammatory, as a treatment for seizures, and more.

CBD Hemp Oil, in the right dosage and form, does not exhibit any psychoactive properties thereby making it an effective treatment option for managing pains and inflammatory-related problems. As there is no fear of addiction with CBD Hemp Oil, its usage is increasing across the world. Moreover, the conventional anti-inflammatory medicines have a lot of harmful side effects which are almost negligible with CBD Oil.

Despite its benefits, a lot more study and research needs to be performed on CBD Hemp Oil and it is, therefore, important to read and garner information about its working, efficiency, side effects, and associated risks before using it. There is definitely a lack of clear-cut regulations and transparency in the cannabis oil industry, making it all the more important for you to arm yourself with the right kind of knowledge in order to make informed choices.

The lack of transparency and the absence of stringent regulation drive unscrupulous people to 'try their luck' in the market in order to earn a quick buck before the 'trend' dies down. Unfortunately, there is a lot of deceptive advertising and misleading marketing rampant in the industry.

Nearly 55% of Americans are believed to be on regular prescription medication. While the percentage is not alarming on the face of it, the fact that prescription medicines are becoming 'normal' to be used by more than half of the population of a country is definitely a cause for concern. The negative effects of prescription medications including 'fixations' or 'addictiveness' can have a debilitating effect on your life.

Unfortunately, other alternative therapeutic options including herbal medicines, homeopathy, Ayurveda, etc., are still not backed by sufficient scientific research to be accepted as viable and effective alternatives.

At this stage, CBD Hemp Oil made its rather silent yet effective entry into the market. Over the course of the last decade, there are plenty of studies that have proven the efficacy of Cannabidiol in the treatment of anxiety, epilepsy, psychotic disorders, stroke rehabilitation, pain, and other disorders.

So, let us get right ahead and find out more about this wonderful CBD Hemp Oil.

Chapter 1: All the Fundamental Information You Need to Know about CBD Hemp Oil

We start this chapter with the most basic information about CBD Hemp Oil.

What is CBD Hemp Oil?

It is extracted typically from Hemp, a fibrous, industrial form of cannabis which sprouts small buds. The tetrahydrocannabinol level in these Hemp buds are very low compared to extracts from Marijuana plants. Tetrahydrocannabinol or THC is the chemical compound that is responsible for people getting high when they smoke cannabis or Marijuana. CBD Hemp Oil is extracted from these buds and then diluted with MCT (Medium-Chain Triglycerides) oil.

There are more than 85 different cannabinoids identified in cannabis and CBD is one of them. After THC, CBD is the most abundantly found cannabinoid in cannabis. However, in Hemp, THC is found only in trace amounts whereas CBD is the dominant component. CBD interacts naturally with our internal systems without being psychotropic, meaning it doesn't get you high. This important biochemical feature of CBD makes it a less controversial and a safer treatment option than medical Marijuana.

Differences between Hemp and Marijuana

Marijuana and Hemp are the most commonly used names for the cannabis plant. The term cannabis brings to mind images of people getting high and stoned. It is hardly associated with useful materials such as military-grade fabric, plant-based plastics, or durable plastic. Yet, the cannabis plant is used for these things as well. So, even though Hemp and Marijuana are forms of the cannabis plant, there are huge differences, which make CBD Hemp Oil more effective and far less harmful than medicinal Marijuana when used for treatments.

Let us study the differences between the two plants under the following four subheadings:

- Genetic Differences
- THC Content
- Cultivation Process
- Legal Status

Genetic Differences – Right through human history, the cannabis plant and its various parts have been used in medicine and in different industries. Early civilizations grew sturdy and tall varieties of cannabis plants to make oils, foods, and textiles (as fabrics and ropes). These cannabis varieties were interbred with other plants with similar characteristics to produce a new variety which we now know as Hemp.

Some varieties of cannabis were identified for their psychoactive properties and were interbred with plants of similar characteristics which were used for medicinal and religious practices. These varieties of cannabis are what we now know as Marijuana. Therefore, Marijuana and Hemp are genetically very different, and are grown in varying agricultural environments too.

Scientists are of the opinion that the genetic interbreeding performed by early human beings resulted in two very distinct cannabis plant types. These two types of cannabis plants are categorized under two separate species; Cannabis sativa and Cannabis indica. CBD Hemp Oil is extracted from the former species, which has negligible psychoactive properties.

Amount of THC – Cannabinoids is the collective name given to some unique compounds found in the cannabis plant. There are many different cannabinoids identified by the scientific community out of which THC or tetrahydrocannabinol, the 'high' inducing compound, is most discussed and well-known.

Marijuana contains a high level of THC whereas the Hemp species contains very little of this psychoactive component. The amount of THC is the primary difference in discerning between Marijuana and Hemp. For instance, in Canada, if the THC level of Hemp is not less than 0.3%, then it is categorized as Marijuana.

Another common cannabinoid found in Hemp and Marijuana species is CBD. The level of CBD is higher than the level of THC in Hemp and this situation is reversed in Marijuana. Multiple research studies have revealed an interesting connection between CBD and THC and that is CBD actually reduces THC's psychoactive effect.

Cultivation Process – As Marijuana and Hemp are cultivated for different purposes, their cultivation processes are also different. Medical cannabis cultivation processes are optimized to produce female flowering plants which yield budding flowers during their flowering stage. Contrarily, Hemp plant cultivation processes are optimized to yield male flowering plants without any flowering buds being produced during their lifecycle. Moreover, centuries of selective breeding of Hemp plants have resulted in a species with very low THC levels and which are characterized by fast-growing tall plants optimized for stalk harvest.

Growing Marijuana is a tricky process that calls for micromanagement of various elements including stable temperature, optimum amount of light, exposure to carbon dioxide, humidity, oxygen levels, and other factors. Marijuana is grown indoors in order to be able to control these factors better. Hemp plants, on the other hand, do not need such detailed monitoring and, therefore, can be grown outdoors to maximize yield and size instead of paying close attention to each plant.

Legal Status – Both Marijuana and Hemp, along with all other varieties of cannabis plants, are not legally cultivable in the US. However, there are many other countries (over 30) that produce Hemp, with China in the lead, followed by Chile and the European Union. Canada is also becoming a popular

Hemp producing nation.

In the US, it is perfectly legal to import Hemp products and this import industry is thriving in the country. Marijuana is outlawed in most of the other countries of the world. While some countries such as Canada and Israel have begun to regulate the production of Marijuana for medicinal purposes with very strict monitoring mechanisms in place, it is still considered a narcotic and its production is illegal in most parts of the world.

These stark differences should clear your mind of the doubts you might have had about the psychoactive properties, if any, in Hemp and Hemp products. Now, let's dig a little deeper and look at the major differences between CBD and THC

Differences between CBD and THC

THC – As already explained, THC is the primary psychoactive component in Marijuana plants that produces the feeling of 'high.' The working of THC is very similar to that of anandamide, a neurotransmitter produced in the brain which is responsible for modulating eating and sleeping habits. Anandamide is also responsible for how a person perceives pain.

THC also exhibits other effects including:

- Relaxation
- Altered sense of hearing, smell, and sight
- Hunger

- Fatigue
- Reduced aggression

In recent years, medical research is proving that medical Marijuana can be effective to treat:

- The side effects of chemotherapy including nausea, reduced appetite, and vomiting
- Multiple sclerosis to improve bladder functioning and spasticity and to reduce spasms and other types of pains
- Glaucoma to reduce eye pressure
- The side effects of AIDS including poor appetite
- Spinal injuries to reduce tremors

CBD – The chemical formulae of CBD and THC are very similar to each other and yet, a slight difference in the arrangement of the THC molecules renders a psychoactive effect to them which is absent in CBD. CBD is available in plentiful in Hemp plants and the lack of the worrisome psychoactive effect makes it a suitable option to treat certain medical conditions. CBD helps to:

- Reduce psychotic symptoms
- Relieve discomforts of nausea and convulsions
- Decrease anxiety
- Decrease inflammation

Research studies have shown promising results of CBD in the treatment of:

- Schizophrenia by reducing psychotic symptoms
- Social anxiety disorder by lowering anxiety levels
- Depression by reducing symptoms of depression

* Cancer side effects by decreasing nausea and pain and improving appetite

The Advantage of CBD over THC for Medical Treatments

THC is categorized as an illegal drug because of its following cognitive-related problems.

* It impairs the user's reasoning and thinking process
* It reduces the user's ability to organize and plan
* It alters decision-making capabilities
* It reduces impulse control

In addition to the above, extended use of THC is known to increase the risks of heart and brain disorders.

CBD, on the other hand, does not impact cognitive abilities negatively. In fact, there are research studies proving the efficacy of CBD in countering the psychoactive effects of THC. Marijuana extracts (even for the sake of medicine) with their high levels of THC and low levels of CBD result in a 'stoned' feeling and Hemp products with less THC and more CBD create an insignificant buzz making CBD Hemp Oil a preferred choice over THC-rich products.

Elements of a Good CBD Hemp Oil Brand

There is no doubt a lack of transparency and clear regulatory control over Hemp products, particularly CBD Hemp Oil. Unfortunately, in such a scenario, the market can and is being used by unscrupulous fly-by-night operators. As expected, the primary aim of people with such low scruples is to make a quick buck and make hay while the sun shines and be ready to run before stringent rules are in place.

As purchasers, we hold a little bit of responsibility to ensure we nip this kind of behavior in the bud by building our knowledge and making sure we don't get taken for a ride. An informed buyer is an essential entity in creating a morally upright marketplace. You need to keep a lookout for the following elements before choosing your brand of CBD Hemp Oil.

Methods of Extractions - The extraction method employed is the primary factor for making CBD Hemp Oil CBD-rich. However, most people do not know that it is important to ask this question. Many companies employ cheap extraction methods involving the use of toxic materials such as hexane, propane, butane, and pentane. These toxic materials are also highly inflammable considering they are all hydrocarbon gases that are found in petroleum.

These toxic solvents are bound to leave behind unsafe residues in the final CBD Hemp Oil. The toxic residue can not only impede the healing process but can also compromise immune functions of an individual. Butane extraction might be efficient and cheap, but the end product is not good. It is important to remember that use of butane and butane products is illegal.

Another form of extraction is through the use of

pharmaceutical-grade, organic ethanol. Some experts say that this form of extraction is good because the process yields optimal CBD and certain residues and toxins of the raw plant are also eliminated. Yet others feel that although the process is Generally Recognized as Safe (GRAS) and the yield of CBD is high, the final product is less potent than it should be.

The third method of extraction is through the use of supercritical carbon dioxide. In this process, carbon dioxide is used in extremely low temperatures and under high pressures to isolate and preserve the CBD Hemp Oil. This process, therefore, is capable of maintaining the purity of the extracted oil. The flipside is that this extraction method is complex, using a lot of processes and equipment making it very expensive. However, you can rest assured about the quality of the end product.

The fourth method of extraction involves the use of coconut oil or olive oil. It is safe and inexpensive too. However, it is perishable and needs to be stored appropriately in a dark, cool place.

Sourcing – The quality of CBD Hemp Oil is highly dependent on where the Hemp was sourced from and what species was used. The climate, soil conditions, the upkeep and maintenance of the farm, and many other factors decide the quality of the sourcing material. The cultivation environment is a critical factor because cannabis plants are basically 'hyperaccumulators' which means they easily absorb contaminants from the soil on which they grow. This characteristic feature of cannabis plants is the reason why they are used as bioremediation agents, a natural way of removing toxicity from the soil.

Therefore, Hemp grown for industrial purposes, in non-food grade environments, is not an ideal raw material for CBD Hemp Oil. If the soil is contaminated with lead, mercury, or other heavy metals, the residual toxic effects will definitely permeate into the Hemp products. It is, therefore, important for you to look for CBD Hemp Oil brands that source their cannabinoids from organic farms that specifically cultivate Hemp for oil extraction purposes. Websites of reputable companies will display the lab results of the various quality tests conducted on their raw materials.

Bioavailabilit*y* – Cannabinoids degrade easily, and their bioavailability reduces over time. There are many cases where CBD Hemp Oil has been found to have zero percent of CBD in it. The reason why bioavailability is an important factor to consider is that the amount of CBD that is effectively absorbed by the human body is a gray area.

Moreover, the first-pass effect is known to affect nearly 90% of CBD consumed. The first-pass test is a term used in drug metabolism which reflects the degradation or alteration levels of a drug that takes place before it enters the general circulatory system of the body. So, a reduced bioavailability could hamper the effectiveness of the CBD Hemp Oil.

This characteristic feature of the drug of any brand is dependent on the overall formulation, the manufacturing process, and the delivery methodology employed (the delivery methods are discussed in another chapter of this book). While it is believed that sublingual and rectal delivery methods are the best for optimum bioavailability, vaping also promises good levels of absorption. Ingestion and topical delivery methods provide lower absorption levels. In such a scenario, maximizing bioavailability is a key factor in the effectiveness of the CBD Hemp Oil.

Some companies adjust the manufacturing/formulation process for increased bioavailability. These methods include reducing the cannabinoids' particle size, immersing the cannabinoid particles in a mixture of natural ingredients that improve absorption, etc. Some companies use synthetic solvents and emulsifiers for improved absorption. Enhanced bioavailability is very tricky to achieve.

If you study the formulation mechanisms of any particular CBD Hemp Oil, you will be in a better position to understand the effectiveness of the processes employed. When you buy CBD Hemp Oil, make sure the label reflects the correct value of active CBD in the product. An ideal combination would be 4 or more parts of CBD to 1 part of THC, which offers optimal results with minimum loss of effectiveness of the stored product over time.

Greenwashing Techniques – Greenwashing or 'window dressing' techniques are employed by many companies to lure people to added benefits from their CBD Hemp Oil. For example, there are brands which boast of the 'superfood moringa' as being an added ingredient in their Hemp Oils. It is important to remember that if ingredients are combined, then the amount, effectiveness, and bioavailability of each of the ingredients in that particular package is going to reduce. It is more prudent, therefore, to stick to the pure ingredient instead.

When the above four conditions are primed in the CBD Hemp Oil product market, then the quality bar is set high. Considering the fact that regulation in this sector is still gray, as users, we need to exercise more caution while making purchases. In addition to caution, making correct and informed choices by the majority of users of CBD Hemp Oil will result in improving the quality standards of the entire CBD market. Make sure you are buying products that offer transparency and fit into the legal framework of the particular geography you belong to.

Chapter 2: Benefits, Side Effects, and Other Variables of CBD Hemp Oil

Before we go into the benefits and side effects of CBD Hemp Oil, let us understand how CBD works in our human system.

How CBD Works in the Human Body

CBD, like all other cannabinoids, needs a receptor in the human body in order to produce and deliver its effects. The human body produces two types of cannabinoids receptors, including CB1 and CB2. While CB1 is found all over the human body, it is more concentrated in the brain than in other parts. The CB1 receptors of the brain are responsible for:

- Coordination and movement
- Pain
- Emotions
- Moods
- Thinking
- Appetite
- Memory

THC attaches itself to the CB1 receptor.

CB2 receptors are prevalent in the immune system and directly affect pain and inflammation. By the way, the human body produces its own cannabinoids. Originally, it was thought that CBD attaches itself to CB2 receptors. However, as more research studies were conducted, and observations made, it seems more likely now that CBD does not attach itself to any of the receptors. Instead, CBD influences the human body to employ its own naturally-produced cannabinoids.

Benefits of CBD

Because of the way CBD works in the human body, scientists and researchers believe that it can offer multiple benefits to mankind.

Natural Anti-Inflammatory Properties – Over-the-counter and prescription drugs are commonly used for pain relief and to relieve stiffness, including the chronic variety. There are experts who believe (based on multiple research studies) that CBD could be a good alternative free of debilitating side-effects. Many scientists opine that CBD, which has little to no psychoactive compounds, can be a new treatment to manage chronic inflammation and pain. There are many oral sprays containing CBD which are approved medications for pain relief in many countries.

Drug Withdrawals and Quitting Smoking – Some studies have revealed promising results in terms of using

CBD to help addicts give up smoking and taking drugs. These studies revealed that people who inhaled CBD ended up smoking a fewer number of cigarettes and needed fewer drug fixes than before. Other studies also revealed that CBD can be an effective treatment to help people de-addict themselves from the use of opioids.

Researchers observed that CBD helps counter certain substance-abuse symptoms such as mood swings, anxiety, insomnia, and pain. While these research studies are still in their nascent stages, the observations show ample promise in this direction.

Brain Disorders Including Epilepsy – There has been a lot of research work undertaken in the use of CBD to treat brain and neuropsychiatric disorders such as epilepsy. Its anti-seizure properties combined with low levels of psychoactive effect make CBD highly suitable for this purpose.

Treatment for epilepsy-linked disorders such as psychiatric diseases, neurodegeneration, and neuronal injury are being studied with the use of CBD and there are some very promising results. Other studies have revealed that CBD could be an effective and safe treatment for schizophrenia because of its ability to behave similarly to certain antipsychotic drugs.

Cancers – Some cancer research studies have revealed that CBD appears to block cancer cells and prevent them from spreading throughout the body. This compound seems to behave in such a way that the growth of cancer cells is not just impeded but cancer cells are also killed. Researchers believe that CBD can be an effective complementary therapy for cancer owing to its low toxicity levels. They believe that CBD should be combined with other existing cancer treatments and synergism of the therapies should be studied further.

Anxiety Disorders – Patients diagnosed with chronic anxiety-related problems are told to avoid taking cannabis because of the presence of THC which only aggravates and worsens existing anxiety disorders and paranoia. However, some studies prove that CBD could be an effective counter-measure to reduce anxiety in certain anxiety disorders. CBD is believed to be useful in countering anxious behaviors and feelings in:

- Post-trauma stress problems
- General anxiety issues
- Obsessive-compulsive disorder
- Social anxiety disorder
- Panic disorder

The prevalent medicines prescribed for these disorders potentially result in very unpleasant side-effects and symptoms such as agitation, drowsiness, sexual dysfunction, headaches, and insomnia. These debilitating side-effects compel many patients to stop taking the medicines. Moreover, some medications such as benzodiazepines are addictive, leading patients to become substance abusers. CBD has not exhibited any kind of adverse side-effects and, therefore, scientists and researchers recommend its use in the treatment of these diseases.

Relieves Nausea – There are studies which prove that cannabinoids, both THC and CBD, can relieve feelings of nausea and vomiting. However, as the psychoactive effects are more in THC than in CBD, the latter is a preferred choice of researchers and scientists. Moreover, very low doses of CBD are sufficient to suppress symptoms of vomiting and nausea.

Type-1 Diabetes - Many research studies have proven that cannabinoids are an effective treatment for insulin-related issues. It has been seen that insulin fasting levels showed a decrease when experimented with CBD. In addition, smaller waist circumference was also noted, which is a direct connection to the onset of Type 1 Diabetes.

Reduction in Acne – This skin condition affects nearly 9% of the world population. The causes are not clearly discernible, and factors include:

- Genetics
- Certain bacteria
- Underlying inflammation
- Excessive production of sebum (an oily secretion produced by sebaceous glands)

Test-tube studies proved the efficacy of CBD Hemp Oil in the treatment of acne because of its ability to decrease sebum production and its anti-inflammatory properties. Additionally, production and release of cytokines, which are inflammatory agents linked to excessive acne, are also kept in check.

Improves the Health of the Heart – There are multiple studies that reveal promising results in the use of CBD oil to improve the functioning and health of the circulatory system and heart. CBD is also seen to be effective in lowering blood pressure, which causes multiple diseases associated with the vascular system such as heart attacks, metabolic issues, and strokes.

People on CBD Hemp Oil have observed lowered blood pressure and improved stress test results. Again, researchers opine that the anxiety- and stress-reducing properties of CBD help in lowering blood pressure. Animal studies have also revealed that CBD can help in the reduction of cell death and inflammation associated with heart diseases because of its powerful stress-reducing and anti-oxidant properties.

Side –Effects of CBD Hemp Oil

Plenty of small-scale studies have been conducted and have proven that CBD Hemp Oil is well-tolerated by most people, though the following side-effects were seen in some people:

Depression and Anxiety – Although CBD is recommended as a treatment for anxiety disorders, there are cases where people have reported anxiety as a side-effect of taking CBD. Any depression occurring as a side-effect could be a result of the incompatibility of the user's brain functioning with the working of CBD. Another reason attributed to this side-effect is the reduced regulation of Central Nervous System (CNS) activation caused by CBD use.

When CNS activation is reduced, most people tend to feel lethargic and tired which could lead to bouts of depression. Most physicians will reduce the dosage of CBD when patients report symptoms of depression. People with a history of psychiatric issues have the highest risk of feeling this side-effect.

Diarrhea – In various clinical trials of CBD in the treatment of psychotic disorders and epilepsy, the most common side-effect reported was diarrhea. Scientists are yet to figure out the reason for this symptom. Many doctors concurrently prescribe other medicines and drugs to counter the effects of diarrhea.

Dry Mouth or Xerostomia – A reported side-effect of CBD is an unpleasant dryness in the mouth. This is considered to be connected to reduced saliva secretion caused by CBD. The cannabinoid receptors CB1 and CB2 are found in the submandibular glands (responsible for saliva production and secretion). When CBD is used, the functioning of the CB1 and CB2 receptors in the submandibular glands are altered, leading to a change in saliva production. This results in a feeling of dryness in the mouth which is also referred to as 'cotton-mouth.'

This drying up of the mouth leads to increased thirst. Staying hydrated is an effective way to counter this side-effect. Also, physicians recommended chewing sugar-free gum to stimulate the salivary glands. A dry mouth is also a great environment for certain harmful bacteria that cause cavities to thrive. Regular visits to the dentist are a must to prevent this problem.

Dizziness, Drowsiness, and Lightheadedness – When higher doses of CBD are taken there appears to be a significant drop in blood pressure which could be the reason for lightheadedness. This side-effect is only temporary, and you simply need to take a cup of coffee or tea to reverse it. Also, this temporary side-effect might go away once the body gets used to the effects of CBD.

While in most cases CBD induces wakefulness, in some cases, especially with high doses, drowsiness can be a result. When this side-effect is in play, it is important not to operate machinery or drive or do anything that requires your focused attention.

Insomnia – Yes, CBD is good for reduced stimulation resulting in improved sleep patterns and restful sleep. Yet, there are people who might be affected by insomnia when they use CBD. Some studies have revealed that certain doses trigger alerting symptoms thereby preventing the onset of restful sleep. A good way to overcome this is to take CBD in the morning or early afternoon instead of at night.

Altered (Reduced) Appetite – While THC is widely known to induce an increase in appetite, people on CBD do not feel ravenously hungry. In fact, one of the side-effects of CBD is reduced appetite. Users of CBD have reported decreased appetite and subsequent weight loss. The theory used to explain this effect is that CBD mitigates the 'liking' or 'wanting' of food. There are no significant side-effects on the central nervous system or changes in vital signs and moods. The side-effect that was most commonly prevalent was fatigue.

Irritability – Again, even though anxiety-reducing effects of CBD mostly help in reducing irritability, there are some people who might find their irritability quotient increased because of CBD use. The reason for this could be that the existing neurochemical condition of the user is incompatible with the workings of CBD. This incompatibility could lead to moodiness and irritability.

However, scientists and experts opine that a more likely cause of irritability is because of decreased activation of neurotransmitters resulting in increased drowsiness, brain fog, and lack of clarity of thought. Some individuals might find these consistent symptoms frustrating which could trigger irritability. People with existing neuro-psychotic symptoms are likely to be at a higher risk of experiencing irritability as a side-effect of CBD use.

Motor Impairment – People whose systems have become accustomed to the regular use of CBD and its effects are not impacted by motor impairment. However, new users, high-dose users, and those who use CBD along with other substances could feel the side-effect of motor impairment. The most common reason for an impaired motor function is a decreased activation of the central nervous system resulting in lowered alertness and sleepiness.

Effect on Hepatic Drug Metabolism – There is a family of liver enzymes that go by the name of cytochrome P450. These enzymes are responsible for the metabolism of nearly all pharmaceutical drugs taken by human beings for various treatments. High doses of CBD can potentially hamper the metabolic activity of this family of enzymes thereby affecting pharmaceutical drug metabolism in our body.

While it is a side-effect of CBD use, many experts do not think it is a bad thing because deactivating P450 enzymes is one of the ways that CBD uses to neutralize the psychoactive effects of THC. In fact, eating a portion of grapefruit has a similar effect on the liver enzymes. It is a minor side effect. Yet, if you are on other medications it is recommended that you take the advice of your physician before consuming CBD Hemp Oil.

Research studies on the uses and benefits of CBD Hemp Oil are still in their nascent stage. A lot more data is required for a wholesome and complete approach to CBD as a therapeutic alternative for various diseases. Tests are not yet carried out for the use of CBD in children.

It is quite difficult to gauge the safety and effectiveness levels of CBD in any brand of CBD Hemp Oil. Speak to your physician before choosing to go with CBD Hemp Oil.

Other Variables that Influence the Occurrence of CBD Side-Effects

There are multiple variables that affect the way CBD Hemp Oil works, including the number and severity of side-effects that it produces. Let us look at some of these variables.

Dosage - The dosage is usually connected to the tolerance levels and to the body weight of the individual. In general, it has been seen that high doses of CBD increase the number and/or severity of side-effects. In fact, some of the side-effects such as tremors in people afflicted with Parkinson's disease are seen only on high doses. No tremors are exhibited when CBD is used in low doses.

Additionally, higher doses of CBD affect the physiology more substantially than lower doses. For example, if you feel slightly drowsy when you are on a low dose of CBD, doubling the dosage is bound to increase the side-effect significantly. Meaning, the side-effects at higher doses are more noticeable and prominent than at lower doses.

Administration – When and how you take your CBD Hemp Oil can influence the number and severity of side-effects that you experience. Whether you take capsules or administer in the sublingual way, whether you take it in the afternoon or late at night, whether you take it after food or before food, etc., affects the way side-effects are exhibited. For example, someone who takes CBD sublingually and at noon will experience very different side-effects from someone who consumes it in capsule form before breakfast.

Empty Vs Full Stomach – Some people might experience the side-effects more prominently when they consume CBD on an empty stomach. Others might feel the side-effects more prominently when consumed on a full stomach. The degree of fullness influences the number and severity of experiencing CBD side-effects.

Delivery Method – There are different ways CBD Hemp Oil can be administered to an individual. This method influences the bioavailability of the ingredient. For example, CBD administered transdermally will result in reduced gastrointestinal issues such as diarrhea, as most of the CBD will be absorbed locally.

Timing – It is a commonly accepted fact among medical professionals that substance and drug use interacts with the internal circadian rhythm. For example, if you take CBD at night, there could be increased drowsiness as it synergizes with your sleeping time. Similarly, if you take CBD in the morning, the effect of drowsiness is far less as it again aligns with the alertness of your body's daytime circadian rhythm.

Specifics in the CBD Hemp Oil – Specific attributes of a particular CBD Hemp Oil affect how side-effects are experienced. For example, a CBD formula with additives and/or contaminants could result in increased side-effects. The specific attributes include:

- Additives
- Contaminants
- Brand
- Purity and Potency
- Sourcing

Additives – A pure form of CBD will have fewer side-effects than one which has added substances such as those that regulate the body's neurochemistry or other phytocannabinoids.

Brand – In the previous chapter, I explained how different companies process CBD Hemp Oil differently which could change the way side-effects are experienced. CBD formulas of brands with excellent quality control over sourcing and the manufacturing processes will have lower side-effects than those brands which have little or no quality control.

Contamination – This element is dependent on the brand of CBD formula you are choosing. The cheaper ones will compromise the quality of sourcing materials and manufacturing processes, resulting in contaminant residuals remaining in the final product. The toxicity of these contaminants could contribute to adverse reactions.

Purity and Potency – A highly potent and pure CBD formula could actually enhance the experience of the side-effects because this potent and pure form will affect the body's physiology significantly more than one which is less pure and potent.

Sourcing – The cultivation process, the harvesting process, and other aspects of the original cannabis plant affect the efficacy of the final CBD formula, which can affect the side-effects experienced as well.

Using Other Substances Concurrently with CBD – Side-effects of CBD Hemp Oil are altered or affected if it is used concurrently with other medication and/or substance abuse. Some medications/substances could exacerbate the side-effects caused by CBD while others could attenuate the side-effects. You must remember to check with your physician and let them know about other prescribed/OTC medications you take.

Duration of Use – The body becomes accustomed to CBD use for a period of time and it is possible that the side-effects could reduce in the long run. In the short term, it is possible that the body gets into an adjustment mode and the side-effects are more pronounced initially. However, it is also possible that in the long-term, new side-effects are displayed as CBD use progresses. As the dosage is increased, new side-effects could be experienced by the user. It is important to know that side-effects of CBD are bound to change over time and the consistency with which you have used it.

Individual Factors – A lot of individual factors including a person's lifestyle, his or her food habits, and other medical conditions could affect the side-effects of CBD Hemp Oil use. Here are a few of the individual factors that play a role in this regard:

Genetics – Genetics are known to play a vital role in the way CBD side-effects are experienced. For example, if the genetic makeup of your body results in a varied form and functioning of the P450 family of enzymes, then the side-effects experienced due to CBD use are different. Genetics that affect the working of cannabinoid receptors could also influence how side-effects are experienced by a person.

Lifestyle – Your diet, sleep, stress levels, and physical fitness levels are known to change the way you feel the side-effects of CBD. A person with a poor diet, lack of restful sleep, or high levels of stress could feel the side-effects of CBD use more than a person who leads a healthy lifestyle.

Medical Conditions – Certain medical conditions enhance side-effects of CBD use. For example, people with Parkinson's are at increased risks of feeling tremors when they are on CBD use. This is because the neurochemical abnormalities of Parkinson's are not compatible with the neurochemical effects of CBD. Keep your medical history and current medical conditions in mind and understand the implications before using CBD.

How to Reduce Side Effects

The following side-effects mitigating methods are known to be very beneficial for users. Again, it is important to consult your physician before you decide.

- Alter the dosage
- Change the administration and delivery mechanisms
- Change the brand of CBD Hemp Oil
- Stop other substance use immediately
- Combine other substances such as an anti-diarrheal agent

- Continue use despite the side-effects to give time to your body to become accustomed to effects of CBD

Despite that rather long narrative on side-effects, you must know that CBD Hemp Oil is known to be well tolerated by most people and severe side-effects or adverse reactions are not common. Being aware of how to mitigate side-effects will prove beneficial for people who want to try the benefits of CBD Oil.

Chapter 3: Application and Delivery Methods, Dosages, and How to Make Your Own CBD Hemp Oil

Before we go into dosages, you need to understand the duration of each dose. How long does each dose remain effective for use in the human body system? This is primarily dependent on the delivery and administrations mechanisms.

Drug Delivery Methods and Duration of Effect

There are four main methods of delivery that can be used to administer CBD Hemp Oil including:

Vaping or Smoking – Here, the CBD Hemp Oil is inhaled through the nostril. This method of inhaling CBD will result in the effect remaining for about 1-4 hours. Vaping is easy and comes in a variety of flavors. The biggest advantage about this delivery method is that people were able to control their smoking urge by inhaling CBD. Vaping CBD Hemp Oil imitates the action of smoking cigarettes without the harmful effects of nicotine. Moreover, vaping CBD Hemp Oil helps in quick and effective absorption.

Sublingual Application – The effect of the sublingual method of delivery lasts for about 1-6 hours. Sublingual CBD is not ingested through the stomach or the digestive system. It is designed for maximum absorption to take place in the mouth itself. Yet, some of it gets swallowed and enters the digestive system too. However, since most of the CBD gets absorbed in the mouth, the sublingual method delivers a faster onset of CBD effects.

Inhalation and sublingual methods deliver the fastest onset of effects but also last for the shortest duration of time. Therefore, you need to have frequent redoes.

Topical Application – The duration of the effects of topically applied CBD is not clearly known. The good thing, however, is that you can apply it liberally without fear of many side-effects. Of course, do a patch test on a small portion of your skin before applying liberally. Wherever you feel pain or irritation, apply CBD Hemp Oil freely. It makes sense to start with a small amount to understand how it works and how long it lasts. Then you can start increasing the amount of application and reapply whenever you need to.

Ingestion – You can ingest CBD Hemp Oil in the form of capsules or even pouring it over the food you eat. A classic example of ingesting CBD Hemp Oil is by eating pot brownies or cannabis brownies. Ingestion takes the longest time for the effect to begin, but lasts longer than other delivery mechanisms. The duration of the ingestion process lasts for any time between 6-8 hours thereby reducing the frequency of consuming the cannabinoid.

Moreover, the duration of the effect of one dose is also dependent on the individual. As it is generally a safe medicine, it makes sense for you to arrive at your own dosage starting from the smallest amount and slowly increasing it while keeping track of the side-effects and the beneficial effects you are experiencing.

General Guidelines for CBD Dosage

To reiterate, every person's dosage requirements are unique and is dependent on many factors including body weight and the severity of the medical condition. Here is a small table that gives you a general guide to CBD daily dosages depending on these two factors:

Severity of Medical Condition	Body Weight Range between 31-60 lbs	Body Weight Range between 61-100 lbs	Body Weight Range between 100-175 lbs	Body Weight Range between 175-250 lbs
Mild Level -1	2mg – 4mg	4mg – 6mg	6mg – 8mg	8mg – 10mg
Mild Level - 2	4mg – 8mg	6mg – 12mg	8mg – 18mg	12mg – 20mg
Medium Level-1	8mg – 12mg	12mg – 18mg	18mg – 24mg	22mg – 30mg

Medium Level-2	12mg – 18mg	18mg – 24mg	24mg – 32mg	32mg – 40mg
Severe Level	18mg – 30mg	24mg- 40mg	32mg – 60mg	42mg – 60mg

Take your weight and start at the lower dosage level. Track both your good and bad experiences for a week or two. Then, gradually increase your dosage to reach the maximum level for your body weight and for the severity of your medical condition. You must wait at least one week for the effects of each dosage change to be adjusted and reflected in your system.

It is important to note at this point that there is no one-size-fits-all dosage schedule. The most effective way of finding the perfect dose for you is through the trial and error method or by experimenting. This is a safe way to do it because there are no fears about a legal overdose with CBD, unlike Marijuana or any other highly psychoactive drug. Even the side-effects are not very common and if they do occur, the severity is mostly mild.

However, when you experiment, it is best to start with the lowest dose recommended for your condition and for your body weight. Then, very gradually, increase the dosage until you reach your desired benefits with minimal side-effects. When you adjust doses, make sure the changes are very small so that the final dosage results are accurate. It is important to reiterate here that at every dosage change, you must give your body at least a week to become adjusted to the changes.

Record your progress. Write down all the details as you

increase CBD doses. These details include:

- The amount of CBD taken
- When taken
- Body weight
- What you ate before and/or after
- Your experiences before taking CBD
- Your experiences after taking CBD

The above is only a general guideline to follow. You must include every relevant thing while you are using CBD. Keep a detailed log and fill it up with data every day so that at any time and point, you can easily find out which elements were beneficial for you and which were not so good for you.

CBD Hemp Oil is presently categorized as a natural supplement as it does not contain any other synthetic chemicals. Reputed and established brands of CBD Hemp Oil ensure that it is extracted directly from the hemp plants under controlled lab environments to ensure the final product meets the natural supplement category requirements.

How to Make Your Own CBD Hemp Oil

Making your own CBD Hemp Oil has multiple benefits. First, it will be cheaper than the branded ones and second, you will be sure that the oil you get is of the purest and the most potent form. You will not be using toxic solvents during the extraction process; you will be able to gauge the quality of the raw material, etc. Some great benefits of making CBD Hemp

Oil at home include:

Quality – You will not have to worry about chemicals and additives in your CBD oil as you have complete control over what is going inside. You are free to choose what ingredients you want and tweak the final product to suit your needs.

Price – Making CBD oil is far cheaper than buying a good brand of oil. The price differences between homemade and commercial CBD Hemp Oil are significant. The cost of store-bought CBD oils is nearly 3-4 times the cost of homemade varieties. You must, of course, be willing to invest your efforts and time in learning different methods of making CBD oil at home.

Potency – As you are in total control of the process and ingredients, you will be able to ensure that you obtain the potency that you want. Moreover, you will have no doubt about the accuracy of the potency too, thereby giving you the flexibility to choose the perfect dosage.

Choosing the Right Strain of Cannabinoid – The following high-CBD strains are good for making the oil at home:

- Charlotte's Web – THC -5% and CBD – 15%
- Pennywise - THC - 9% and CBD – 9%
- Haley's Comet - THC - 8% and CBD - 8%
- Harlequin - THC - 5% and CBD - 15%
- Cannatonic - THC- 1% and CBD - 15%,

Here are a couple of simple recipes you can use to make CBD Hemp Oil at home.

Recipe #1 (with ground buds)

Ingredients and Equipment:

- Ground buds – 30 g Or
- Dried, ground trim or shake – 60-100g
- Any food-safe alcohol
- Ceramic or glass mixing bowl
- A really fine strainer such as nylon stockings, or a fine sieve, or cheesecloth
- Catchment container
- Double boiler
- Plastic syringe, funnel, silicon spatula, and a wooden spoon

Procedure:

Keep all your ingredients and equipment on a clean, dry work area. Put the buds in the ceramic bowl and cover it fully with alcohol. Stir the mixture for about 3-5 minutes until all the resin is separated. The bowl should be big enough to comfortably hold the ground cannabis buds and the required alcohol.

Using any of the strainers mentioned above, filter this mixture and catch the first extraction in the catchment container ensuring you squeeze out as much liquid as you can. Use another batch of alcohol and repeat this stirring and filtering process to get as much compound from the plant extracts as possible.

Now, pour this filtered solution into the double boiler. Heat it until bubbles appear. Allow the bubbling to continue without increasing the temperature until the alcohol evaporates completely. To keep the temperature more or less constant, you can either adjust the heat source or turn on and turn off the heater appropriately while keeping the solution bubbling gently for about half an hour.

It is important to keep stirring the mixture to prevent it from getting very hot. When the alcohol evaporates completely, mix the solution thoroughly. Remember to scrape off the bottom of the bowl with the wooden or silicon spatula. You can quickly transfer this warm liquid into dry, dark, airtight containers to prevent it from thickening further. Alternately, you can store the liquid in the plastic syringes.

This CBD Hemp Oil extraction process is very safe and suitable for ingestion. The extracted oil will be quite thick, and you can dilute it with any vegetable oil or olive oil or coconut oil while it is still warm. This can serve as excellent topical ointments.

Recipe #2 (with CBD concentrate crystals)

Step 1: Add 1 cup of canola, coconut or olive oil to a pot. Place it on the stove and turn it onto the lowest heat and allow the oil to simmer gently.

Step 2: Crush 1 gm of CBD isolate crystals (which you can buy at medical stores) and put it into the pot of simmering oil. CBD concentrates which are the most potent and purest form of CBD are available in different forms including wax or crystals (for vaping purposes) or CBD tinctures.

Step 3: Now, stir this mixture gently until the CBD concentrate dissolves completely in the oil. Now, turn off the stove and allow the mixture to cool down. Pour the cooled CBD oil in an airtight jar. You can store this oil at room temperature.

You can alter the potency and strength of the oil by changing the amount of CBD crystals. To find the amount of CBD in one teaspoon, you will need to divide the amount of CBD crystals you used by the amount of oil you used (in teaspoon measure). 1 cup of oil is equivalent to 48 teaspoons of oil.

So, to illustrate this calculation, suppose you used 600 mg of CBD crystals to dissolve in 1 cup of oil, then you will get 48 teaspoons of CBD oil with 12.5 mg of CBD in each teaspoon. You can safely keep the oil obtained through this method for up to 2 months. If you refrigerate it, you can extend the shelf-life even further.

Other Differences between Homemade and Manufactured CBD Hemp Oil

Other differences between homemade and manufactured CBD Hemp Oils can be understood by the following elements:

Extraction – Large brands and companies use professional extractors for the extraction process which results in a full-spectrum CBD oil containing a range of cannabinoids from the hemp plant including, of course, CBD. Homemade CBD is only CBD. While the benefits and effects are more or less the same in both kinds of extraction processes, the full-spectrum CBD oil interacts and activates the entire cannabinoid system of our body which can be good or bad depending on your needs.

Ingredients – The ingredients that go into homemade CBD oil are entirely in your control, thereby preventing the addition of harmful solvents, chemicals, and additives. Professional brands' manufacturing process invariably involves the use of chemicals in some way or the other with residual effects being transferred to the final product. Although the set of ingredients are mentioned on the label, one can never be completely sure. It would be great if you get the CBD Oil tested at an independent third-party lab to ensure quality.

Packaging – Homemade oils are stored in used (but cleaned and dried) jars or bottles whereas commercial oils come in neat, comfortable packaging that is easy to use too.

While the convenience of store-bought CBD Hemp Oil is great, making your own has amazing benefits. Considering that the research work on the effectiveness and side-effects of CBD is still in the nascent stage, ensuring quality is a great way to prevent falling into traps laid by unscrupulous brands and companies. That said, there are many companies that promise quality and deliver it too. You need to do your research and identify the places where you can shop for good-quality CBD Hemp Oil.

Chapter 4: Research Studies on CBD Hemp Oil

The reason for the rising popularity of CBD is definitely its therapeutic capabilities over a wide range of diseases and disorders. Researchers are continuing their work on understanding and identifying the potential of this cannabinoid.

Overall Safety of CBD

A safety and side-effects review was published in June 2017 by scientists of a German University (https://www.ncbi.nlm.nih.gov/pmc/articles/PMC5569602/). This review work was based on a huge collection of existing information from other research work done on the safety level of CBD. This review was basically done to organize and synthesize vast amounts of existing data into a comprehensive report on the safety and side-effects aspects of CBD. The following conclusions were drawn:

- CBD is safe for human use
- There is a lot more research work to be done on its therapeutic effects to treat epilepsy and other psychotic disorders
- The most common side-effects caused by CBD are diarrhea, tiredness, and appetite changes
- The side-effects of CBD were less compared to the side-effects of conventional prescription drugs
- CBD can be an effective supplementary therapy

CBD for Treating Drug-Resistant Seizures

A research paper published in August 2017 by a group of Spanish scientists threw light on the effectiveness of CBD to treat drug-resistant seizures, also referred to as refractory epilepsy (https://www.neurologia.com/articulo/2016573/eng). A group of 15 people were given CBD for periods ranging from 30 days to a year. The following encouraging results were observed:

- About 40% of patients reported reduced frequency of seizures
- In 27% of patients, the seizures disappeared completely
- 60% of the patients were able to have better control over some of their seizures
- Many patients reported improvement in language skills, behavior, sleep patterns, and eating habits.
- 100% of patients reported improved moods
- The most common side-effects reported were fatigue and drowsiness

CBD for Treating Seizures in Children

CBD was tested for its effectiveness in the treatment of seizures in children with Dravet Syndrome, a rare genetic epileptic disorder that usually develops in the first year itself. It can lead to developmental disabilities in the afflicted child. Traditional medicines do not help much because this is a form of refractory epilepsy.

A pool of 120 young adults and children were involved in the double-blind, placebo-controlled research program which included a 14-week treatment plan. The following findings were recorded:

(https://www.nejm.org/doi/full/10.1056/NEJMoa1611618?q uery=featured_home)

- Convulsive seizures in children treated with CBD reduced from 12.4% to 5.9% whereas the placebo group reported only a 0.8% decrease. However, non-convulsive seizure rates did not change. 5% of the CBD-treated group became free of seizures compared to 0% from the placebo group.
- Side-effects including fever and vomiting were significantly increased in the CBD-treated group of children. Yet, 62% of the children in the CBD group reported significant improvement in their condition, whereas only 34% of the placebo-treated children reported improvements.
- While the adverse side-effects are an issue, the overwhelmingly positive response to CBD shows immense promise in treating children with Dravet Syndrome.

CBD to Overcome Fear of Public Speaking

This research was conducted by a group of scientists and the report was published in May 2017 (https://www.ncbi.nlm.nih.gov/pmc/articles/PMC5425583/). The study involved 60 male and female participants between the ages of 18 and 35. Participants were divided into five group who were randomly administered a placebo or CBD in doses of 900mg or 300mg or 100mg) or clonazepam, a traditional drug prescribed for panic disorders. The results were as follows:

- Clonazepam gave the best results as it reduces anxiety in a more sedating manner than CBD or the placebo.
- However, the 300mg dose of CBD showed a significant reduction in anxiety levels in the post-speech phase.

- The main focus of the study was to observe how varied dosages of CBD worked in reducing anxiety.
- These findings reiterate the importance of getting the CBD dosage right

CBD to Treat High Blood Pressure

A study to check the effectiveness of CBD to lower high blood pressure was conducted by a group of scientists and the report was published in June 2015 (https://insight.jci.org/articles/view/93760)

This placebo-controlled, double-blind study involved nine healthy male participants (volunteers) who were randomly administered a placebo or 600mg CBD. The volunteers' cardiovascular systems were monitored, and changes were recorded. Stress tests such as math problems without the use of calculators were given to them and their cardiovascular systems were monitored. It was found that CBD reduced stroke volume as well as the systolic blood pressure at rest. The study also found that CBD was able to blunt the response of blood pressure to stressful situations.

The Psychoactive Properties of CBD

The close connection between CBD and THC is one of the primary reasons for medical professionals' reticence in using the former for medical therapies. A study to combat this idea was conducted by a group of scientists and researchers (https://www.liebertpub.com/doi/10.1089/can.2017.0034) at Indiana University and the report was published in September 2017. This study also compared earlier studies, where CBD was tested in in-vitro lab conditions for psychoactive effects. In these tests, CBD was converted into

THC, which prompted the negative psychoactive notions against CBD. The results read as follows:

The scientists noted that in in-vitro conditions, it might be possible for CBD to convert to THC. However, many studies have proven that in in-vitro conditions, the conversion of CBD to THC is not evidenced or suggested. Researchers in this study have cautioned scientists and medical professionals from misinterpreting and misrepresenting extrapolated figures of results and observations from research studies.

Effects of CBD on Anxiety Levels and Emotional Stimuli

This study was conducted to check the effects of CBD on anxiety levels of users (https://www.ncbi.nlm.nih.gov/pmc/articles/PMC5569582/). This placebo-controlled, double-blind research program involved 38 participants who were randomly administered varying doses of CBD or a placebo. Their anxiety levels and their responses to emotional stimuli were monitored by giving them different tasks, including those that involved situations resulting in social rejections or changes in emotional facial expressions.

The tasks covered a rollercoaster of emotions for volunteers and it was noted that their responses were not affected by either placebo or varying doses of CBD. These observations clearly showed that CBD does not affect emotions or moods and does not have any effect on the users' anxiety levels.

The good thing about this result is that CBD does not alter an individual's perception of the world, and the bad thing is that CBD may not be such a great choice of therapy for treating anxiety. Of course, there are other studies which offer contrasting results that CBD can effectively calm down anxious emotions and, therefore, can be a potential therapy for anxiety disorders.

CBD to Treat Schizophrenia-like Cognitive Impairment

The conventional antipsychotic drugs prescribed for schizophrenia have far fewer benefits compared to the severe adverse effects. CBD with its antipsychotic and inflammatory properties was seen as a possible alternative to conventional drugs. A group of scientific reviewers undertook a systematic review   of (https://www.ncbi.nlm.nih.gov/pubmed/27884751) existing scientific literature on the subject.

This group reviewed studied 27 articles published over a period of 26 years and came to the conclusion that CBD has the potential to improve cognitive function in patients afflicted with cognitive impairment as in cases of schizophrenia, Alzheimer's disease, neurological disorders such as epilepsy, and neuroinflammatory conditions such as fibromyalgia.

CBD as an Alternative to Addiction-Prone Prescription Drugs for Pain

This survey was undertaken by research scientists to find an effective alternative for pain instead of heavy and addictive medication that is being used currently. https://www.liebertpub.com/doi/10.1089/can.2017.0012. There were 2897 CBD-rich-cannabis users who participated in this survey. Of the participants who were using opiates about six months before starting off on CBD, the following findings were reported:

- 97% agreed that they were able to reduce their dependency on opiates after taking CBD
- 81% agreed that CBD by itself improved their symptoms better than combining it with opioids

The survey participants also said that the effectiveness of CBD was as good as other conventional medication without the adverse side-effects.

CBD to Treat Liver Injury

A study, published in September 2017, revealed that it is possible to use CBD to heal liver injuries caused by chronic alcoholism.
(https://www.ncbi.nlm.nih.gov/pmc/articles/PMC5608708/)

CBD was administered to mice and to human blood samples that were fed with alcohol. It was noticed that CBD administration helped in reducing the level of liver enzymes as well as liver triglycerides. CBD also facilitated the reduction in fat droplet accumulation. The study also noted the following observations:

- CBD improved liver metabolism that was impaired by alcohol consumption
- It reduced abnormal lipid retention

With these observations, researchers concluded that CBD can be a potential therapy for alcohol-induced liver problems such as steatosis, inflammation, and oxidative stress.

It is important to remember that the results and observations made from the above studies are fairly broad in nature and a lot more work needs to be done. Yet, these are not the first or the last set of studies done to test the effectiveness of using CBD to treat a plethora of health issues, ranging from serious disorders to simple pains and inflammations.

The good thing about these studies is the fact that a lot of them are using information from earlier studies and are taking off from where the previous stopped, resulting in a positive progression. Continued research work will help us to gain more knowledge about the benefits and side-effects of CBD.

Chapter 5: Success Stories of People Who Used CBD Hemp Oil

While research studies are great and give us a lot of scientific insight into the workings of CBD Hemp Oil, the personal success stories of people who have used it and been directly benefited by it are more encouraging. Here is a list of success stories that I have compiled for your benefit: (please note that the names of some of the people have been changed to protect their privacy).

CBD for Pain Relief

A bad road accident in 2014 left Nell Smith of Colorado completely shattered, both physically and mentally. Managing the agonizing pain associated with three herniated disks turned his life completely awry. He couldn't get back to his job as a garage mechanic despite being highly skilled. He was on multiple conventional pills including morphine, Oxycontin, and many more NSAIDs (both OTC and prescribes).

However, nothing worked for him and the pain simply got worse. Moreover, the nasty and unpleasant adverse effects of the medication left him tired and drained. He finally decided to try CBD Hemp Oil after reading up on its effectiveness to control pain and inflammation. It was recommended to him by his friend who had used CBD to manage a backache. He used a well-known brand of CBD Hemp Oil and found it reduced the pain from his lower back rapidly. The best part was that his mood improved considerably, even as his tolerance to pain got better.

Another success story is that of Kevin Cochran who works as a bartender. In an unforeseen accident, a glass bottle cut through his hand, severing the right median nerve. He needed a fast-acting pain relief option as he couldn't afford to stay off work for a very long time. He used CBD Hemp Oil in three forms including vaping, topical application, and ingestion. The combination worked wonders for Kevin and he got his much-need fast-relief action and was able to get back to work quickly.

CBD to Manage Multiple Sclerosis Symptoms

David Booth from Texas was diagnosed with multiple sclerosis when he was 20 years of age way back in 2006. He continued to fight the battle against the disease with the symptoms of fatigue, headaches, spasms, and insomnia, enhancing the difficulty of leading a normal life.

Like most people, David too tried a host of prescription drugs to control and manage these symptoms to little or no avail. Like Nell, David was more overcome with the severe adverse reactions of the prescription drugs rather than benefitting from reduced symptoms. Finally, his doctor told him about CBD Hemp Oil and he decided to give it a try.

After consultations with his physician, David started using the oil in the morning after waking up and at night before going to bed. He arrived at a dosage that was perfect for him after multiple trial and errors. Now, he is completely off all the prescription drugs except the medication for MS. What made him the happiest was the complete absence of any kind of side-effects.

CBD for Migraines and Menstrual Pains

Shelley Merali, a 47-year-old mother of two, had been suffering from migraines for over 20 years now. Her menstrual cycles were painful too with her migraines increasing in intensity during those times of the month. The problems aggravated even further by her menopause. She used to take Advil and Excedrin for her pains, many times, over six a day. This medication left her jittery throughout the day and her migraines and pains hardly reduced.

One of her friends suggested vaping low-THC, high-CBD cannabis through a vape pen. In about a week, Shelley found relief. The intensity and frequency of her migraines reduced considerably and within a fortnight, they almost disappeared. Moreover, her menstrual cycle pains also became less. She tells her friends that she has found a wonder-drug that keeps pain at bay without her feeling stoned.

CBD for Skin Rashes

CBD-infused salves treat burns and wounds very well. Here is a classic example of how CBD came to the help of Stella Rubens, who had a genetic skin disorder called Hailey-Hailey. This disease is characterized by inflammation, blisters, and rashes that are brought on by a weak skin-cell development mechanism. Enzyme mutation is known to be the primary reason for the impaired skin-cell development process.

Hailey-Hailey manifests itself usually during the adolescent stage and the condition worsens with age and the skin development functioning gets increasingly impaired. The condition is associated with the lack of elasticity in the skin because of abnormalities in the affected skin cells as well as the surrounding collagen, resulting in weakened and cracked skin. Stella Rubens was suffering a lot from her teenage days from this malady. Steroids are commonly prescribed by doctors for this condition.

As expected, steroids with their nasty side-effects made Stella's already-brittle skin condition worse. Her doctor recommended the use of CBD-infused salves to heal blisters and rashes. These salves also contained multiple beneficial herbs, oils, and beeswax along with CBD oil. This salve has anti-bacterial properties too and was very effective to manage symptoms of Hailey-Hailey. The CBD oil helps counteract the flair-ups caused by steroids too. Stella's life changed so much for the better since she started using CBD to manage skin inflammations.

CBD Tinctures for Seizures

CBD in the tincture form facilitates fast therapeutic action and is highly effective for seizure patients. Betty Shire, a 30-year-old lady living in Tennessee, was diagnosed with Multiple Sclerosis in 2014. Since then, she has been experiencing 8-10 seizures a year. She tried eight different seizure medicines and none of them were effective. Around January 2017, she started using CBD along with the prescribed seizure medicines. She is yet to experience even a single seizure since then. She uses CBD tincture of a popular and established brand. Her dosage ranges between 2-3 500 mg CBD drops thrice a day. She also drizzles coconut oil-diluted CBD oil over her dishes during breakfast, lunch, and dinner. She arrived at this dosage after multiple experiments and to ensure that her body feels the effects of CBD oil 24/7.

CBD for Sound Sleep as Well as for Alertness

CBD is known to help give users sound sleep in the night without the hangover associated with psychoactive drugs. Jordan Mayo of Denver is a very busy 35-year-old man juggling a jewelry business and a musical instrument store. In his spare time, he is part of a local band too, where he plays the guitar and sings. The overactive lifestyle made sleep very difficult in the night for Jordan and he kept getting up frequently. His friend recommended CBD to help him overcome insomnia. When he started using CBD, Jordan realized that its effect was doubly beneficial and here's how.

This busy man needs to be super alert and active during the day and get a restful night's sleep too. CBD works perfectly for Jordan as the effects are aligned with the natural circadian rhythm of the user. So, his morning dose of around 150 mg of CBD oil keeps him alert right through the day, giving him the needed strength to multitask and get everything done. The nightly dose helps him to sleep soundly, allowing him to get up in the morning fresh and alert without feeling hungover.

CBD for Anxiety and Depression

Anxiety disorders are a rising cause of mental health concern across the US. Nearly half of the people who have anxiety disorders also suffer from depression. Sharon O'Donnell was one of the many who went through the problems of anxiety and depression. She was affected so much that she would be scared to leave her home because of panic attacks. She suffered from suicidal tendencies as well.

In January 2015, she started ingesting CBD in the form of

capsules. After consulting with her physician and through trial and error, Sharon arrived at the following dosage: 150 mg of CBD taken twice a day in the form of pills. She now goes around feeling very confident of herself and believes that CBD changed the way her brain worked, resulting in eliminating feelings of catastrophe and anxiety from her system.

In fact, there are CBD-infused medicinal baths that help in relaxation as well. The bath soaks contain 99% CBD isolates and are combined with sea salt extracts for reducing muscle aches, essential oils for skin nourishment and aromatherapy. A ritual bath using this soak is bound to lower stress and decrease anxiety levels for everyone. For Sharon, this ritual bath has become part of her daily therapy.

Customizing CBD Dosage is Essential

Each one of us is different and our needs are different too. There are no standards for CBD dosage except to remain within the minimum and maximum limits given in the guideline dosage table in this book. Here is a story of Michelle Brown's CBD dosage customizing method. Michelle had painful headaches that used to subside a little when she took prescription drugs. As soon as the effect of the drug reduced, the headaches would return.

Michelle's husband then had a bad accident and was crippled irreversibly. He became bedridden and she was his sole caregiver. The stress of this situation made her anxious and depressed, which increased the frequency and severity of her headaches. She was flustered and frustrated. A gentleman in her husband's support group told her about CBD which he was using himself.

Michelle did a lot of research on CBD oil and also consulted her physician. She decided to start with tinctures. On the first day, she tried micro-dosing with a 1000mg CBD tincture bottle. Her headache disappeared completely when she came to her third drop and Michelle thought she had found her perfect dose. However, her headache returned half an hour later.

So, the next day, she started with three drops in the morning. However, the headache returned again in about an hour. She realized that three drops continuously didn't work for her. On the third day, she spaced out her three drops equally throughout the day and found herself free from headaches when she woke up on the morning of the fourth day of her trial.

This just goes to show that dosages have to be adjusted and the effects tracked before you find one that is perfect for your body physiology. Michelle was lucky that she found her 'sweet spot' in three days' time. It is possible that it will take longer than this. Just be patient with yourself, make detailed notes, and persist in your trial and error method, and sooner rather than later you will find your 'sweet spot' too.

These real-life success stories and the negligible side-effects are sufficient reasons to take advantage of the benefits of CBD Hemp Oil. Start small, increase gradually, make detailed recordings, and you will find the ideal CBD therapy for your specific need.

Conclusion

There is no doubt that a lot of research still needs to be done before the scientific community clearly understands CBD Hemp Oil. And the needed work is going on too. However, there is little doubt that CBD's psychoactive properties are nowhere as much as that of THC. Therefore, the chances of getting into substance abuse with CBD are very, very low.

Not only THC, even prescription drugs of conventional medicine are known to lead users to substance abuse. There is no such fear with using CBD Oil. Another point in favor of CBD oil is that it is gaining in popularity and this would not be possible if people were not happy with the efficacy of the product.

The one element I would like to reiterate in the concluding note is to do a considerable amount of research before deciding your course of action. Take all factors into account, including your physical and mental condition and speak to your physician too. Do not get carried away by cheap prices. Identify a reputable company, research their processes and other manufacturing aspects and purchase the CBD Hemp Oil product only when you are satisfied with the quality.